MW00339081

# THE TYPE 1 DIABETES COOKBOOK 2021

Easy and Healthy Diabetic Diet Recipes for Type 1 Diabetes

# Table of Contents

7

Additionally, the information in the following pages is intended only for informational purposes and should thus be thought of as universal. As befitting its nature, it is presented without assurance regarding its prolonged validity or interim quality. Trademarks that are mentioned are done without written consent and can in no way be considered an endorsement from the trademark holder.

# Introduction

Type 1 diabetes (T1D) occurs when the body is unable to produce insulin, a hormone produced by the pancreas. Although the exact cause is unknown, it is believed to be a combination of genetics and environment. Today, an estimated 1.25 million people live with T1D in the United States, and 40,000 people are diagnosed every year. T1D results when the body's immune system attacks and destroys its own cells; in this case, it kills the healthy insulin-producing cells. Without insulin from these cells, the body is unable to help sugar (glucose) enter the cells to provide energy.

I wish there were another answer, but currently, management of T1D always requires insulin. Regardless of any changes you implement in your diet, vitamin intake, or lifestyle, if you are diagnosed with T1D, you will need insulin.

Insulin is an amazing hormone produced by the pancreas. The pancreas works to regulate blood sugar, or glucose, levels. It works like this: You eat something, your body digests the foods you eat, and some of that food (mostly carbohydrates but also protein and some fats) converts to glucose, which is the body's primary source of energy. Once glucose is released into the bloodstream, the pancreas responds and releases insulin, which helps move the glucose into our cells for energy. With type 1 diabetes, an outside source of insulin needs to be delivered to do the job; this is typically achieved by injecting insulin or by using an insulin pump.

T1D differs from T2D in that in type 2, the body actually produces insulin, but often the insulin that is produced does not work effectively. With T2D, oral medication, non-insulin injectables, and lifestyle changes are the primary treatments

The following dietary guidelines will be helpful to anyone with type 1 diabetes.

**Aim for a balanced diet.** Seek out carbohydrates that are full of fiber, such as whole grains, fresh fruits, and nonprocessed vegetables. Include fish three times per week, as well as lean meats and calcium-rich protein sources, like tofu and milk. Use healthy fats, such as monounsaturated fat—these include olive and avocado oils, seeds, nuts, and nut butters. Enjoy caffeine and alcohol in moderation, limit simple sugars, and drink plenty of water.

**Understand insulin action and meal timing.** If you're unclear about how to time your insulin and meals, please discuss this with your diabetes educator. To be effective, insulin and meal timing need to coordinate; this will also help prevent low and high blood sugars.

**Read labels.** Reading labels is one of the most important things you can do in the grocery store. Become a label-reading pro! In doing so, try not to fall for any misleading claims, like those that read "sugar-free" or "no added sugar." Look at serving sizes and total grams of carbohydrates. Aim for products with at least 3 grams of fiber per 100 calories and less than 5 grams of sugar.

**Include healthy proteins.** Protein is essential for cell growth and repair. Include healthy, lean proteins, such as fish, tofu, or poultry. You will not take insulin to cover for protein portions unless you are eating unusually large amounts compared to your regular intake.

**Carry a simple form of sugar.** Keep portable snacks with you, like juice boxes, sports drinks, hard candy, jelly beans, dried fruit, honey, or glucose tablets or gels. You may need them to treat low blood sugars. Even with the best of intentions, low blood sugars can occur, so be prepared by keeping simple sugars on hand.

**If you drink alcohol, eat when you do.** Surprisingly, alcohol can lower blood sugars. It's always a good idea to eat some form of carbohydrates when you have a cocktail. Talk to your doctor about the best way to manage food, alcohol, and insulin.

**Drink plenty of water.** Is there any diet that doesn't advocate water? This diet is no different. In fact, it may be even more important for people with diabetes, since people with diabetes are at higher risk for dehydration. Don't wait until you're thirsty, and try to drink 8 to 10 glasses of water throughout the day. Also, limit beverages containing caffeine! Aim for less than 250 milligrams of caffeine daily.

# Chapter 1.   Food List For Type 1 Diabetes

Treatment through the dietary approach is considered the most effective and logical today. Many of the fatal health conditions are now treated only with a well-oriented health diet plan. The same is true for diabetes. With few adjustments in the routine menu, a patient can maintain his glucose levels without the use of medicines. To make this idea work, we need to cut down the direct or high sources of glucose in the food. Here is the complete list of the items which can be taken on a diabetes-friendly diet.

## What to Have on A Type 1 Diabetic Diet

### Vegetables

Fresh vegetables never cause harm to anyone. So, adding a meal full of vegetables is the best shot for all diabetic patients. But not all vegetables contain the same number of macronutrients. Some vegetables contain a high amount of carbohydrates, so those are not suitable for a diabetic diet. We need to use vegetables which contain a low amount of carbohydrates.

1. Cauliflower
2. Spinach
3. Tomatoes
4. Broccoli
5. Lemons
6. Artichoke

7. Garlic
8. Asparagus
9. Spring onions
10. Onions
11. Ginger etc.

## Meat

Meat is not on the red list for the diabetic diet. It is fine to have some meat every now and then for diabetic patients. However certain meat types are better than others. For instance, red meat is not a preferable option for such patients. They should consume white meat more often whether it's seafood or poultry. Healthy options in meat are:

1. All fish, i.e., salmon, halibut, trout, cod, sardine, etc.
2. Scallops
3. Mussels
4. Shrimp
5. Oysters etc.

## Fruits

Not all fruits are good for diabetes. To know if the fruit is suitable for this diet, it is important to note its sugar content. Some fruits contain a high number of sugars in the form of sucrose and fructose, and those should be readily avoided. Here is the list of popularly used fruits which can be taken on the diabetic diet:

1. Peaches

2. Nectarines
3. Avocados
4. Apples
5. Berries
6. Grapefruit
7. Kiwi Fruit
8. Bananas
9. Cherries
10. Grapes
11. Orange
12. Pears
13. Plums
14. Strawberries

## Nuts and Seeds

Nuts and seeds are perhaps the most enriched edibles, and they contain such a mix of macronutrients which can never harm anyone. So diabetic patients can take the nuts and seeds in their diet without any fear of a glucose spike.

1. Pistachios
2. Sunflower seeds
3. Walnuts
4. Peanuts
5. Pecans
6. Pumpkin seeds
7. Almonds
8. Sesame seeds etc.

## Grains

Diabetic patients should also be selective while choosing the right grains for their diet. The idea is to keep the amount of starch as minimum as possible. That is why you won't see any white rice in the list rather it is replaced with more fibrous brown rice.

1. Quinoa
2. Oats
3. Multigrain
4. Whole grains
5. Brown rice
6. Millet
7. Barley
8. Sorghum
9. Tapioca

## Fats

Fat intake is the most debated topic as far as the diabetic diet is concerned. As there are diets like ketogenic, which are loaded with fats and still proved effective for diabetic patients. The key is the absence of carbohydrates. In any other situation, the fats are as harmful to people with diabetes as any normal person. Switching to unsaturated fats is a better option.

1. Sesame oil
2. Olive oil
3. Canola oil
4. Grapeseed oil
5. Other vegetable oils
6. Fats extracted from plant sources.

## Diary

Any dairy product which directly or indirectly causes a glucose rise in the blood should not be taken on this diet. other than those, all products are good to use. These items include:

1. Skimmed milk
2. Low-fat cheese
3. Eggs
4. Yogurt
5. Trans fat-free margarine or butter

## Sugar Alternatives

Since ordinary sugars or sweeteners are strictly forbidden on a diabetic diet. There are artificial varieties that can add sweetness without raising the level of carbohydrates in the meal. These substitutes are:

1. Stevia
2. Xylitol
3. Natvia
4. Swerve
5. Monk fruit
6. Erythritol

Make sure to substitute them with extra care. The sweetness of each sweetener is entirely different from the table sugar, so add each in accordance with the intensity of their flavor. Stevia is the sweetest of them, and it should be used with more care. In place of 1 cup of sugar, a teaspoon of stevia is enough. All other sweeteners are more or less similar to sugar in their intensity of sweetness.

## Foods to Avoid

Knowing a general scheme of diet helps a lot, but it is equally important to be well familiar with the items which have to be avoided. With this list, you can make your diet a hundred% sugar-free. There are many other food items which can cause some harm to a diabetic patient as the sugars do. So, let's discuss them in some detail here.

### 1. Sugars

Sugar is a big NO-GO for a diabetic diet. Once you have diabetes, you would need to say goodbye to all the natural sweeteners which are loaded with carbohydrates. They contain polysaccharides which readily break into glucose after getting into our body. And the list does not only include table sugars but other items like honey and molasses should also be avoided.

1. White sugar
2. Brown sugar
3. Confectionary sugar
4. Honey
5. Molasses
6. Granulated sugar

It is not easy to suddenly stop using sugar. Your mind and your body, will not accept the abrupt change. It is recommended to go for a gradual change. It means start substituting it with low carb substitutes in a small amount, day by day.

## 2. High Fat Dairy Products

Once you have diabetes, you may get susceptible to a number of other fatal diseases including cardiovascular ones. That is why experts strictly recommend avoiding high-fat food products, especially dairy items. The high amount of fat can make your body insulin resistant. So even when you take insulin, it won't be of any use as the body will not work on it.

## 3. Saturated Animal Fats

Saturated animal fats are not good for anyone, whether diabetic or normal. So, better avoid using them in general. Whenever you are cooking meat, try to trim off all the excess fat. Cooking oils made out of these saturated fats should be avoided. Keep yourself away from any of the animal origin fats.

## 4. High Carb Vegetables

Vegetables with more starch are not suitable for diabetes. These veggies can increase the carbohydrate levels of food. So, omit these from the recipes and enjoy the rest of the less starchy vegetables. Some of the high carb vegetables are:

1. Potatoes
2. Sweet potatoes
3. Yams etc.

## 5. Cholesterol Rich Ingredients

Bad cholesterol or High-density Lipoprotein has the tendency to deposit in different parts of the body and obstructs the flow of blood and the regulation of hormones. That is why food items having high bad cholesterol are not good for diabetes. Such things should be replaced with the ones with low cholesterol.

## 6. High Sodium Products

Sodium is related to hypertension and blood pressure. Since diabetes is already the result of a hormonal imbalance in the body, in the presence of excess sodium—another imbalance—a fluid imbalance may occur which a diabetic body cannot tolerate. It adds up to already present complications of the disease. So, avoid using food items with a high amount of sodium. Mainly store packed items, processed foods, and salt all contain sodium, and one should avoid them all. Use only the 'Unsalted' variety of food products, whether it's butter, margarine, nuts, or other items.

## 7. Sugary Drinks

Cola drinks or other similar beverages are filled with sugars. If you had seen different video presentations showing the amount of the sugars present in a single bottle of soda, you would know how dangerous those are for diabetic patients. They can drastically increase the amount of blood glucose level within 30 minutes of drinking. Fortunately, there are many sugar-free varieties available in the drinks which are suitable for diabetic patients.

## 8. Sugar Syrups and Toppings

A number of syrups available in the markets are made out of nothing but sugar. Maple syrup is one good example. For a diabetic diet, the patient should avoid such sugary syrups and also stay away from the sugar-rich toppings available in the stores. If you want to use them at all, trust yourself and prepare them at home with a sugar-free recipe.

## 9. Sweet Chocolate and Candies

For diabetic patients, sugar-free chocolates or candies are the best way out. Other processed chocolate bars and sweets are extremely damaging to their health, and all of these should be avoided. You can try and prepare healthy bars and candies at home with sugar-free recipes.

## 10.  Alcohol

Alcohol has the tendency to reduce the rate of our metabolism and take away our appetite, which can render a diabetic patient into a very life-threatening condition. Drink in a very small amount cannot harm the patient, but the regular or constant intake of alcohol is bad for health and glucose levels.

# Chapter 2.   Breakfast

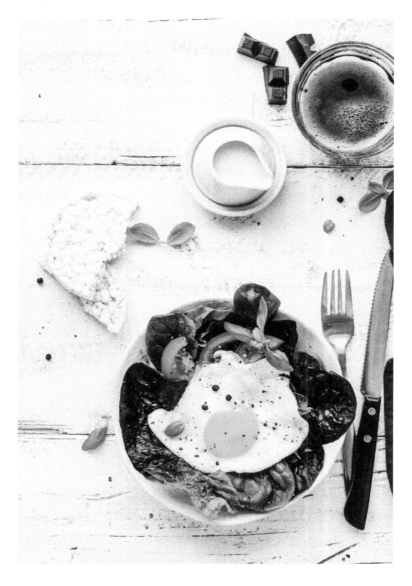

# 1. Pineapple & Strawberry Smoothie

**Preparation Time:** 7 minutes

**Cooking Time:** 0 minute

**Servings:** 2

**Ingredients:**

- 1 cup strawberries
- 1 cup pineapple, chopped
- ¾ cup almond milk
- 1 tablespoon almond butter

**Directions:**

1. Add all ingredients to a blender.
2. Blend until smooth.
3. Add more almond milk until it reaches your desired consistency.
4. Chill before serving.

**Nutrition:**

255 Calories

39g Carbohydrate

5.6g Protein

## 2. Green Smoothie

**Preparation Time:** 12 minutes

**Cooking Time:** 0 minute

**Servings:** 2

**Ingredients:**

- 1 cup vanilla almond milk (unsweetened)
- ¼ ripe avocado, chopped
- 1 cup kale, chopped
- 1 banana
- 2 teaspoons honey
- 1 tablespoon chia seeds
- 1 cup ice cubes

**Directions:**

1. Combine all the ingredients in a blender.
2. Process until creamy.

**Nutrition:**

343 Calories

14.7g Carbohydrate

5.9g Protein

# 3. Spicy Jalapeno Popper Deviled Eggs

**Preparation Time:** 5 minutes

**Cooking Time:** 5 minutes

**Servings:** 4

Ingredients

- 4 large whole eggs, hardboiled
- 2 tablespoons Keto-Friendly mayonnaise
- ¼ cup cheddar cheese, grated
- 2 slices bacon, cooked and crumbled
- 1 jalapeno, sliced

## Directions:

1. Cut eggs in half, remove the yolk and put them in bowl
2. Lay egg whites on a platter
3. Mix in remaining ingredients and mash them with the egg yolks
4. Transfer yolk mix back to the egg whites
5. Serve and enjoy!

## Nutrition:

Calories: 176

Fat: 14g

Carbohydrates: 0.7g

Protein: 10g

# 4. Lovely Porridge

**Preparation Time:** 15 minutes

**Cooking Time:** Nil

**Servings:** 2

Ingredients

- 2 tablespoons coconut flour
- 2 tablespoons vanilla protein powder
- 3 tablespoons Golden Flaxseed meal
- 1 and 1/2 cups almond milk, unsweetened
- Powdered erythritol

**Directions:**

1. Take a bowl and mix in flaxseed meal, protein powder, coconut flour and mix well
2. Add mix to the saucepan (placed over medium heat)
3. Add almond milk and stir, let the mixture thicken
4. Add your desired amount of sweetener and serve
5. Enjoy!

**Nutrition:**

Calories: 259

Fat: 13g

Carbohydrates: 5g; Protein: 16g

# 5. Salty Macadamia Chocolate Smoothie

**Preparation Time:** 5 minutes

**Cooking Time:** Nil

**Servings:** 1

Ingredients

- 2 tablespoons macadamia nuts, salted
- 1/3 cup chocolate whey protein powder, low carb
- 1 cup almond milk, unsweetened

**Directions:**

1. Add the listed ingredients to your blender and blend until you have a smooth mixture
2. Chill and enjoy it!

**Nutrition:**

Calories: 165

Fat: 2g

Carbohydrates: 1g

Protein: 12g

# 6. Basil and Tomato Baked Eggs

**Preparation Time:** 10 minutes

**Cooking Time:** 15 minutes

**Servings:** 4

Ingredients

- 1 garlic clove, minced
- 1 cup canned tomatoes
- ¼ cup fresh basil leaves, roughly chopped
- 1/2 teaspoon chili powder
- 1 tablespoon olive oil
- 4 whole eggs
- Salt and pepper to taste

**Directions:**

1. Preheat your oven to 375 degrees F
2. Take a small baking dish and grease with olive oil
3. Add garlic, basil, tomatoes chili, olive oil into a dish and stir
4. Crackdown eggs into a dish, keeping space between the two
5. Sprinkle the whole dish with salt and pepper
6. Place in oven and cook for 12 minutes until eggs are set and tomatoes are bubbling
7. Serve with basil on top
8. Enjoy!

**Nutrition**:

Calories 235

Fat: 16g

Carbohydrates7g

Protein: 14g

# 7. Cinnamon and Coconut Porridge

**Preparation Time:** 5 minutes

**Cooking Time:** 5 minutes

**Servings:** 4

Ingredients

- 2 cups of water
- 1 cup 36% heavy cream
- 1/2 cup unsweetened dried coconut, shredded
- 2 tablespoons flaxseed meal
- 1 tablespoon butter
- 1 and 1/2 teaspoon stevia
- 1 teaspoon cinnamon
- Salt to taste
- Toppings as blueberries

**Directions:**

1. Add the listed ingredients to a small pot, mix well
2. Transfer pot to stove and place it over medium-low heat
3. Bring to mix to a slow boil
4. Stir well and remove the heat
5. Divide the mix into equal servings and let them sit for 10 minutes
6. Top with your desired toppings and enjoy!

**Nutrition**:

Calories: 171

Fat: 16g

Carbohydrates: 6g

Protein: 2g

# 8. An Omelet of Swiss chard

**Preparation Time:** 5 minutes

**Cooking Time:** 5 minutes

**Servings:** 4

Ingredients

- 4 eggs, lightly beaten
- 4 cups Swiss chard, sliced
- 2 tablespoons butter
- 1/2 teaspoon garlic salt
- Fresh pepper

**Directions:**

1. Take a non-stick frying pan and place it over medium-low heat
2. Once the butter melts, add Swiss chard and stir cook for 2 minutes
3. Pour egg into the pan and gently stir them into Swiss chard
4. Season with garlic salt and pepper
5. Cook for 2 minutes
6. Serve and enjoy!

**Nutrition:**

Calories: 260

Fat: 21g

Carbohydrates: 4g; Protein: 14g

# Chapter 3.  Lunch

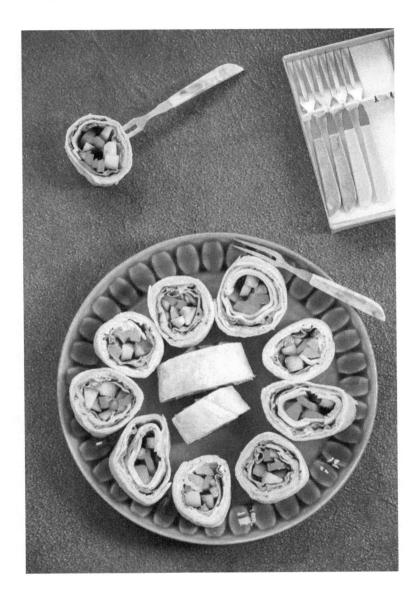

# 9. Berry Apple Cider

**Preparation Time:** 15 minutes

**Cooking Time:** 3 hours

**Servings:** 3

Ingredients

- 4 cinnamon sticks, cut into 1-inch pieces
- 1½ teaspoons whole cloves
- 4 cups apple cider
- 4 cups low-calorie cranberry-raspberry juice drink
- 1 medium apple

Direction

1. To make the spice bag, cut out a 6-inch square from double thick, pure cotton cheesecloth. Put in the cloves and cinnamon, then bring the corners up, tie it closed using a clean kitchen string that is pure cotton.
2. In a 3 1/2- 5-quart slow cooker, combine cranberry-raspberry juice, apple cider, and the spice bag.
3. Cook while covered over low heat setting for around 4-6 hours or on a high heat setting for 2-2 1/2 hours.

4. Throw out the spice bag. Serve right away or keep it warm while covered on friendly or low-heat setting up to 2 hours, occasionally stirring. Garnish each serving with apples (thinly sliced).

## Nutrition

89 Calories

22g Carbohydrate

19g Sugar

## 10. Brunswick Stew

**Preparation Time:** 10 minutes

**Cooking Time:** 45 minutes

**Servings:** 3

Ingredients

- 4 ounces diced salt pork
- 2 pounds chicken parts
- 8 cups water
- 3 potatoes, cubed
- 3 onions, chopped
- 1 (28 ounce) can whole peeled tomatoes
- 2 cups canned whole kernel corn
- 1 (10 ounce) package frozen lima beans
- 1 tablespoon Worcestershire sauce
- 1/2 teaspoon salt
- 1/4 teaspoon ground black pepper

Direction

1. Mix and boil water, chicken and salt pork in a big pot on high heat. Lower heat to low. Cover then simmer until chicken is tender for 45 minutes.

2. Take out chicken. Let cool until easily handled. Take meat out. Throw out bones and skin. Chop meat to bite-sized pieces. Put back in the soup.

3. Add ground black pepper, salt, Worcestershire sauce, lima beans, corn, tomatoes, onions and potatoes. Mix well. Stir well and simmer for 1 hour, uncovered.

## Nutrition

368 Calories

25.9g Carbohydrate

27.9g Protein

# 11.  Buffalo Chicken Salads

**Preparation Time:** 7 minutes

**Cooking Time:** 3 hours

**Servings:** 5

Ingredients

- 1½ pounds chicken breast halves
- ½ cup Wing Time® Buffalo chicken sauce
- 4 teaspoons cider vinegar
- 1 teaspoon Worcestershire sauce
- 1 teaspoon paprika
- 1/3 cup light mayonnaise
- 2 tablespoons fat-free milk
- 2 tablespoons crumbled blue cheese
- 2 romaine hearts, chopped
- 1 cup whole grain croutons
- ½ cup very thinly sliced red onion

Direction

1. Place chicken in a 2-quarts slow cooker. Mix Worcestershire sauce, 2 teaspoons of vinegar and Buffalo sauce in a small bowl; pour over chicken. Dust with paprika. Close and cook for 3 hours on low-heat setting.

2. Mix the leftover 2 teaspoons of vinegar with milk and light mayonnaise together in a small bowl at serving time; mix in blue cheese.

While chicken is still in the slow cooker, pull meat into bite-sized pieces using two forks.

3. Split the romaine among 6 dishes. Spoon sauce and chicken over lettuce. Pour with blue cheese dressing then add red onion slices and croutons on top.

## Nutrition

274 Calories

11g Carbohydrate

2g Fiber

## 12. Cacciatore Style Chicken

**Preparation Time:** 10 minutes

**Cooking Time:** 4 hours

**Servings:** 6

Ingredients

- 2 cups sliced fresh mushrooms
- 1 cup sliced celery
- 1 cup chopped carrot
- 2 medium onions, cut into wedges
- 1 green, yellow, or red sweet peppers
- 4 cloves garlic, minced
- 12 chicken drumsticks
- ½ cup chicken broth
- ¼ cup dry white wine
- 2 tablespoons quick-cooking tapioca
- 2 bay leaves
- 1 teaspoon dried oregano, crushed
- 1 teaspoon sugar
- ½ teaspoon salt
- ¼ teaspoon pepper
- 1 (14.5 ounce) can diced tomatoes
- 1/3 cup tomato paste

- Hot cooked pasta or rice

Direction

1. Mix garlic, sweet pepper, onions, carrot, celery and mushrooms in a 5- or 6-qt. slow cooker. Cover veggies with the chicken. Add pepper, salt, sugar, oregano, bay leaves, tapioca, wine and broth.
2. Cover. Cook for 3–3 1/2 hours on high-heat setting.
3. Take chicken out; keep warm. Discard bay leaves. Turn to high-heat setting if using low-heat setting. Mix tomato paste and undrained tomatoes in. Cover. Cook on high-heat setting for 15 more minutes. **Servings:** Put veggie mixture on top of pasta and chicken.

## Nutrition

324 Calories

7g Sugar:

35g Carbohydrate

# 13. Carnitas Tacos

**Preparation Time:** 10 minutes

**Cooking Time:** 5 hours

**Servings:** 4

Ingredients

- 3 to 3½-pound bone-in pork shoulder roast
- ½ cup chopped onion
- 1/3 cup orange juice
- 1 tablespoon ground cumin
- 1½ teaspoons kosher salt
- 1 teaspoon dried oregano, crushed
- ¼ teaspoon cayenne pepper
- 1 lime
- 2 (5.3 ounce) containers plain low-fat Greek yogurt
- 1 pinch kosher salt
- 16 (6 inch) soft yellow corn tortillas, such as Mission® brand
- 4 leaves green cabbage, quartered
- 1 cup very thinly sliced red onion
- 1 cup salsa (optional)

Direction

1. Take off meat from the bone; throw away bone. Trim meat fat. Slice meat into 2 to 3-inch pieces; put in a slow cooker of 3 1/2 or 4-quart in size. Mix in cayenne, oregano, salt, cumin, orange juice and onion.

2. Cover and cook for 4 to 5 hours on high. Take out meat from the cooker. Shred meat with two forks. Mix in enough cooking liquid to moisten.

3. Take out 1 teaspoon zest (put aside) for lime crema, squeeze 2 tablespoons lime juice. Mix dash salt, yogurt, and lime juice in a small bowl.

4. Serve lime crema, salsa (if wished), red onion and cabbage with meat in tortillas. Scatter with lime zest.

**Nutrition**

301 Calories

28g Carbohydrate

7g Sugar

# 14. Chicken Chili

**Preparation Time:** 6 minutes

**Cooking Time:** 1 hour

**Servings:** 4

Ingredients

- 3 tablespoons vegetable oil
- 2 cloves garlic, minced
- 1 green bell pepper, chopped
- 1 onion, chopped
- 1 stalk celery, sliced
- 1/4-pound mushrooms, chopped
- 1-pound chicken breast
- 1 tablespoon chili powder
- 1 teaspoon dried oregano
- 1 teaspoon ground cumin
- 1/2 teaspoon paprika
- 1/2 teaspoon cocoa powder
- 1/4 teaspoon salt
- One pinch of crushed red pepper flakes
- One pinch ground black pepper
- 1 (14.5 oz) can tomatoes with juice
- 1 (19 oz) can kidney beans

Direction

1. Fill two tablespoons of oil into a big skillet and heat it at moderate heat. Add mushrooms, celery, onion, bell pepper, and garlic, sautéing for 5 minutes. Put it to one side.

2. Insert the leftover one tablespoon of oil into the skillet. At high heat, cook the chicken until browned and its exterior turns firm. Transfer the vegetable mixture back into the skillet.

3. Stir in ground black pepper, hot pepper flakes, salt, cocoa powder, paprika, oregano, cumin, and chili powder. Continue stirring for several minutes to avoid burning. Pour in the beans and tomatoes, lead the entire mixture to a boiling point, and then adjust the setting to low heat. Place a lid on the skillet and leave it simmering for 15 minutes. Uncover the skillet and leave it simmering for another 15 minutes.

## Nutrition

308 Calories

25.9g Carbohydrate

29g Protein

## 15.  Chicken Vera Cruz

**Preparation Time:** 7 minutes

**Cooking Time:** 10 hours

**Servings:** 5

Ingredients

- One medium onion, cut into wedges
- 1-pound yellow-skin potatoes
- Six skinless, boneless chicken thighs
- 2 (14.5 oz.) cans of no-salt-added diced tomatoes
- 1 fresh jalapeño chili pepper
- Two tablespoons Worcestershire sauce
- One tablespoon chopped garlic
- One teaspoon dried oregano, crushed
- ¼ teaspoon ground cinnamon
- 1/8 teaspoon ground cloves
- ½ cup snipped fresh parsley
- ¼ cup chopped pimiento-stuffed green olives

Direction

1. Put the onion in a 3 1/2- or 4-quart slow cooker. Place chicken thighs and potatoes on top. Drain and discard juices from a can of tomatoes. Stir undrained and drained tomatoes, cloves, cinnamon, oregano, garlic,

Worcestershire sauce and jalapeño pepper together in a bowl. Pour over all in the cooker.

2. Cook with a cover for 10 hours on low-heat setting.

3. To make the topping: Stir chopped pimiento-stuffed green olives and snipped fresh parsley together in a small bowl. Drizzle the topping over each serving of chicken.

## Nutrition

228 Calories

9g Sugar

25g Carbohydrate

# 16.  Chicken and Cornmeal Dumplings

**Preparation Time:** 8 minutes

**Cooking Time:** 8 hours

**Servings:** 4

Ingredients

Chicken and Vegetable Filling

- 2 medium carrots, thinly sliced
- 1 stalk celery, thinly sliced
- 1/3 cup corn kernels
- ½ of a medium onion, thinly sliced
- 2 cloves garlic, minced
- 1 teaspoon snipped fresh rosemary
- ¼ teaspoon ground black pepper
- 2 chicken thighs, skinned
- 1 cup reduced sodium chicken broth
- ½ cup fat-free milk
- 1 tablespoon all-purpose flour

Cornmeal Dumplings

- ¼ cup flour
- ¼ cup cornmeal
- ½ teaspoon baking powder
- 1 egg white

- 1 tablespoon fat-free milk

- 1 tablespoon canola oil

Direction

1. Mix 1/4 teaspoon pepper, carrots, garlic, celery, rosemary, corn, and onion in a 1 1/2 or 2-quart slow cooker. Place chicken on top. Pour the broth atop mixture in the cooker.

2. Close and cook on low-heat for 7 to 8 hours.

3. If cooking with the low-heat setting, switch to high-heat setting (or if heat setting is not available, continue to cook). Place the chicken onto a cutting board and let to cool slightly. Once cool enough to handle, chop off chicken from bones and get rid of the bones. Chop the chicken and place back into the mixture in cooker. Mix flour and milk in a small bowl until smooth. Stir into the mixture in cooker.

4. Drop the Cornmeal Dumplings dough into 4 mounds atop hot chicken mixture using two spoons. Cover and cook for 20 to 25 minutes more or until a toothpick come out clean when inserted into a dumpling. (Avoid lifting lid when cooking.) Sprinkle each of the serving with coarse pepper if desired.

5. Mix together 1/2 teaspoon baking powder, 1/4 cup flour, a dash of salt and 1/4 cup cornmeal in a medium bowl. Mix 1 tablespoon canola oil, 1 egg white and 1 tablespoon fat-free milk in a small bowl. Pour the egg mixture into the flour mixture. Mix just until moistened.

**Nutrition**

369 Calories; 9g Sugar; 47g Carbohydrate

## 17.  Chicken and Pepperoni

**Preparation Time:** 4 minutes

**Cooking Time:** 4 hours

**Servings:** 5

Ingredients

- 3½ to 4 pounds meaty chicken pieces
- 1/8 teaspoon salt
- 1/8 teaspoon black pepper
- 2 ounces sliced turkey pepperoni
- ¼ cup sliced pitted ripe olives
- ½ cup reduced-sodium chicken broth
- 1 tablespoon tomato paste
- 1 teaspoon dried Italian seasoning, crushed
- ½ cup shredded part-skim mozzarella cheese (2 ounces)

Direction

1. Put chicken into a 3 1/2 to 5-qt. slow cooker. Sprinkle pepper and salt on the chicken. Slice pepperoni slices in half. Put olives and pepperoni into the slow cooker. In a small bowl, blend Italian seasoning, tomato paste and chicken broth together. Transfer the mixture into the slow cooker.

2. Cook with a cover for 3-3 1/2 hours on high.

3. Transfer the olives, pepperoni and chicken onto a serving platter with a slotted spoon. Discard the cooking liquid. Sprinkle cheese over the chicken. Use foil to loosely cover and allow to sit for 5 minutes to melt the cheese.

## Nutrition

243 Calories

1g Carbohydrate

41g Protein

## 18. Chicken and Sausage Gumbo

**Preparation Time:** 6 minutes

**Cooking Time:** 4 hours

**Servings:** 5

Ingredients

- 1/3 cup all-purpose flour
- 1 (14 ounce) can reduced-sodium chicken broth
- 2 cups chicken breast
- 8 ounces smoked turkey sausage links
- 2 cups sliced fresh okra
- 1 cup water
- 1 cup coarsely chopped onion
- 1 cup sweet pepper
- ½ cup sliced celery
- 4 cloves garlic, minced
- 1 teaspoon dried thyme
- ½ teaspoon ground black pepper
- ¼ teaspoon cayenne pepper
- 3 cups hot cooked brown rice

Direction

1. To make the roux: Cook the flour upon a medium heat in a heavy medium-sized

saucepan, stirring periodically, for roughly 6 minutes or until the flour browns. Take off the heat and slightly cool, then slowly stir in the broth. Cook the roux until it bubbles and thickens up.

2. Pour the roux in a 3 1/2- or 4-quart slow cooker, then add in cayenne pepper, black pepper, thyme, garlic, celery, sweet pepper, onion, water, okra, sausage, and chicken.

3. Cook the soup covered on a high setting for 3 - 3 1/2 hours. Take the fat off the top and serve atop hot cooked brown rice.

## Nutrition

230 Calories

3g Sugar

19g Protein

## 19. Chicken, Barley, and Leek Stew

**Preparation Time:** 10 minutes

**Cooking Time:** 3 hours

**Servings:** 2

Ingredients

- 1-pound chicken thighs
- 1 tablespoon olive oil
- 1 (49 ounce) can reduced-sodium chicken broth
- 1 cup regular barley (not quick-cooking)
- 2 medium leeks, halved lengthwise and sliced
- 2 medium carrots, thinly sliced
- 1½ teaspoons dried basil or Italian seasoning, crushed
- ¼ teaspoon cracked black pepper

Direction

1. In the big skillet, cook the chicken in hot oil till becoming brown on all sides. In the 4-5-qt. slow cooker, whisk the pepper, dried basil, carrots, leeks, barley, chicken broth and chicken.

2. Keep covered and cooked over high heat setting for 2 – 2.5 hours or till the barley softens. As you wish, drizzle with the parsley or fresh basil prior to serving.

**Nutrition**

248 Calories

6g Fiber

27g Carbohydrate

## 20. Cider Pork Stew

**Preparation Time:** 9 minutes

**Cooking Time:** 12 hours

**Servings:** 3

Ingredients

- 2 pounds pork shoulder roast
- 3 medium cubed potatoes
- 3 medium carrots
- 2 medium onions, sliced
- 1 cup coarsely chopped apple
- ½ cup coarsely chopped celery
- 3 tablespoons quick-cooking tapioca
- 2 cups apple juice
- 1 teaspoon salt
- 1 teaspoon caraway seeds
- ¼ teaspoon black pepper

Direction

1. Chop the meat into 1-in. cubes. In the 3.5-5.5 qt. slow cooker, mix the tapioca, celery, apple, onions, carrots, potatoes and meat. Whisk in pepper, caraway seeds, salt and apple juice.

2. Keep covered and cook over low heat setting for 10-12 hours. If you want, use the celery leaves to decorate each of the servings.

## Nutrition

244 Calories

5g Fiber

33g Carbohydrate

# 21.  Creamy Chicken Noodle Soup

**Preparation Time:** 7 minutes

**Cooking Time:** 8 hours

**Servings:** 4

Ingredients

- 1 (32 fluid ounce) container reduced-sodium chicken broth
- 3 cups water
- 2½ cups chopped cooked chicken
- 3 medium carrots, sliced
- 3 stalks celery
- 1½ cups sliced fresh mushrooms
- ¼ cup chopped onion
- 1½ teaspoons dried thyme, crushed
- ¾ teaspoon garlic-pepper seasoning
- 3 ounces reduced-fat cream cheese (Neufchâtel), cut up
- 2 cups dried egg noodles

Direction

1. Mix together the garlic-pepper seasoning, thyme, onion, mushrooms, celery, carrots, chicken, water and broth in a 5 to 6-quart slow cooker.

2. Put cover and let it cook for 6-8 hours on low-heat setting.

3. Increase to high-heat setting if you are using low-heat setting. Mix in the cream cheese until blended. Mix in uncooked noodles. Put cover and let it cook for an additional 20-30 minutes or just until the noodles become tender.

## Nutrition

170 Calories

3g Sugar

2g Fiber

## 22.  Cuban Pulled Pork Sandwich

**Preparation Time:** 6 minutes

**Cooking Time:** 5 hours

**Servings:** 5

Ingredients

- 1 teaspoon dried oregano, crushed
- ¾ teaspoon ground cumin
- ½ teaspoon ground coriander
- ¼ teaspoon salt
- ¼ teaspoon black pepper
- ¼ teaspoon ground allspice
- 1 2 to 2½-pound boneless pork shoulder roast
- 1 tablespoon olive oil
- Nonstick cooking spray
- 2 cups sliced onions
- 2 green sweet peppers, cut into bite-size strips
- ½ to 1 fresh jalapeño pepper
- 4 cloves garlic, minced
- ¼ cup orange juice
- ¼ cup lime juice

- 6 heart-healthy wheat hamburger buns, toasted
- 2 tablespoons jalapeño mustard

Direction

1. Mix allspice, oregano, black pepper, cumin, salt, and coriander together in a small bowl. Press each side of the roast into the spice mixture. On medium-high heat, heat oil in a big non-stick pan; put in roast. Cook for 5mins until both sides of the roast is light brown, turn the roast one time.

2. Using a cooking spray, grease a 3 1/2 or 4qt slow cooker; arrange the garlic, onions, jalapeno, and green peppers in a layer. Pour in lime juice and orange juice. Slice the roast if needed to fit inside the cooker; put on top of the vegetables covered or 4 1/2-5hrs on high heat setting.

3. Move roast to a cutting board using a slotted spoon. Drain the cooking liquid and keep the jalapeno, green peppers, and onions. Shred the roast with 2 forks then place it back in the cooker. Remove fat from the liquid. Mix half cup of cooking liquid and reserved vegetables into the cooker. Pour in more cooking liquid if desired. Discard the remaining cooking liquid.

4. Slather mustard on rolls. Split the meat between the bottom roll halves. Add avocado on top if desired. Place the roll tops to sandwiches.

## Nutrition

379 Calories; 32g Carbohydrate; 4g Fiber

# 23. Lemony Salmon Burgers

**Preparation Time:** 10 Minutes

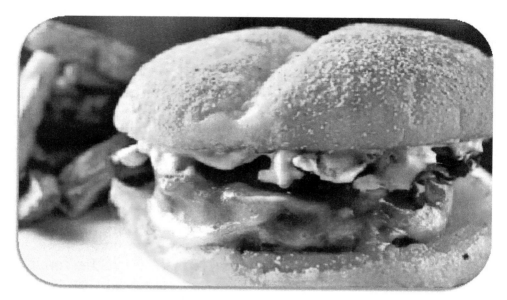

**Cooking Time:** 10 Minutes

**Servings:** 4

Ingredients

- 2 (3-oz) cans boneless, skinless pink salmon
- 1/4 cup panko breadcrumbs
- 4 tsp. lemon juice
- 1/4 cup red bell pepper
- 1/4 cup sugar-free yogurt
- 1 egg
- 2 (1.5-oz) whole wheat hamburger toasted buns

Directions

1. Mix drained and flaked salmon, finely-chopped bell pepper, panko breadcrumbs.

2. Combine 2 tbsp. cup sugar-free yogurt, 3 tsp. fresh lemon juice, and egg in a bowl. Shape mixture into 2 (3-inch) patties, bake on the skillet over medium heat 4 to 5 Minutes per side.

3. Stir together 2 tbsp. sugar-free yogurt and 1 tsp. lemon juice; spread over bottom halves of buns.

4. Top each with 1 patty, and cover with bun tops.

5. This dish is very mouth-watering!

**Nutrition:**

Calories 131 / Protein 12 / Fat 1 g / Carbs 19 g

## 24. Caprese Turkey Burgers

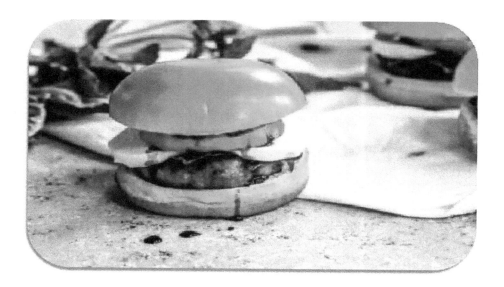

Preparation Time 10 Minutes

**Cooking Time:** 10 Minutes

**Servings:** 4

Ingredients

- 1/2 lb. 93% lean ground turkey
- 2 (1,5-oz) whole wheat hamburger buns (toasted)
- 1/4 cup shredded mozzarella cheese (part-skim)
- 1 egg
- 1 big tomato
- 1 small clove garlic
- 4 large basil leaves

- 1/8 tsp. salt
- 1/8 tsp. pepper

Directions

1. Combine turkey, white egg, Minced garlic, salt, and pepper (mix until combined);

2. Shape into 2 cutlets. Put cutlets into a skillet; cook 5 to 7 Minutes per side.

3. Top cutlets properly with cheese and sliced tomato at the end of cooking.

4. Put 1 cutlet on the bottom of each bun.

5. Top each patty with 2 basil leaves. Cover with bun tops.

**Nutrition**:

Calories 180 / Protein 7 g / Fat 4 g / Carbs 20 g

## 25.  Pasta Salad

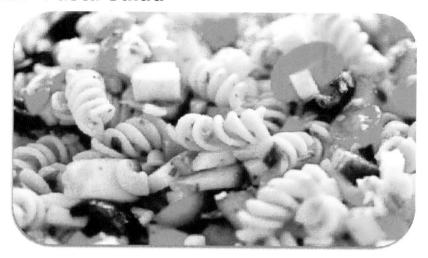

**Preparation Time:** 15 Minutes

**Cooking Time:** 15 Minutes

**Servings:** 4

Ingredients

- 8 oz. whole-wheat pasta
- 2 tomatoes
- 1 (5-oz) pkg spring mix
- 9 slices bacon
- 1/3 cup mayonnaise (reduced-fat)
- 1 tbsp. Dijon mustard
- 3 tbsp. apple cider vinegar
- 1/4 tsp. salt
- 1/2 tsp. pepper

Directions

1. Cook pasta.

2. Chilled pasta, chopped tomatoes and spring mix in a bowl.

3. Crumble cooked bacon over pasta.

4. Combine mayonnaise, mustard, vinegar, salt and pepper in a small bowl.

5. Pour dressing over pasta, stirring to coat.

**Nutrition**:

Calories 200 / Protein 15 g / Fat 3 g / Carbs 6 g

# Chapter 4.  Dinner

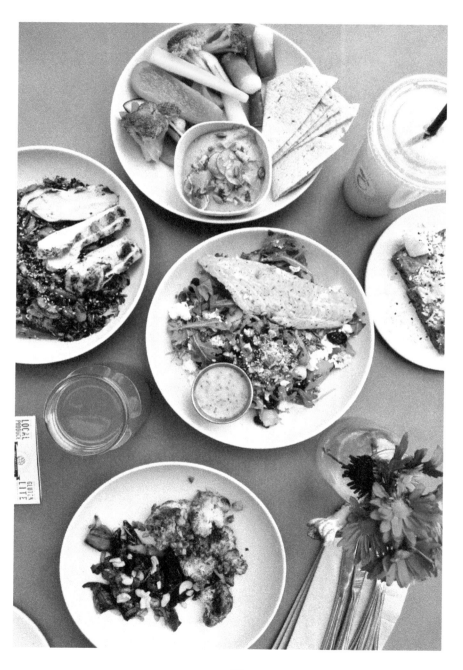

## 26.  Tuna Sweet Corn Casserole

**Preparation Time:** 10 minutes

**Cooking Time:** 35 Minutes

**Servings:** 2

**Ingredients:**

- 3 small tins of tuna
- 0.5lb sweet corn kernels
- 1lb chopped vegetables
- 1 cup low sodium vegetable broth
- 2tbsp spicy seasoning

**Directions:**

1. Mix all the ingredients in your Instant Pot.
2. Cook on Stew for 35 minutes.
3. Release the pressure naturally.

**Nutrition**:  Calories: 300;Carbs: 6 ;Sugar: 1 ;Fat: 9 ;Protein: ;GL: 2

## 27. Lemon Pepper Salmon

**Preparation Time:** 10 minutes

**Cooking Time:** 10 Minutes

**Servings:** 4

**Ingredients:**

- 3 tbsps. ghee or avocado oil
- 1 lb. skin-on salmon filet
- 1 julienned red bell pepper
- 1 julienned green zucchini
- 1 julienned carrot
- ¾ cup water
- A few sprigs of parsley, tarragon, dill, basil or a combination
- 1/2 sliced lemon
- 1/2 tsp. black pepper
- ¼ tsp. sea salt

**Directions:**

1. Add the water and the herbs into the bottom of the Instant Pot and put in a wire steamer rack making sure the handles extend upwards.
2. Place the salmon filet onto the wire rack, with the skin side facing down.
3. Drizzle the salmon with ghee, season with black pepper and salt, and top with the lemon slices.
4. Close and seal the Instant Pot, making sure the vent is turned to "Sealing".

5. Select the "Steam" setting and cook for 3 minutes.
6. While the salmon cooks, julienne the vegetables, and set aside.
7. Once done, quick release the pressure, and then press the "Keep Warm/Cancel" button.
8. Uncover and wearing oven mitts, carefully remove the steamer rack with the salmon.
9. Remove the herbs and discard them.
10. Add the vegetables to the pot and put the lid back on.
11. Select the "Sauté" function and cook for 1-2 minutes.
12. Serve the vegetables with salmon and add the remaining fat to the pot.
13. Pour a little of the sauce over the fish and vegetables if desired.

**Nutrition**: Calories 296, Carbs 8g, Fat 15 g, Protein 31 g, Potassium (K) 1084 mg, Sodium (Na) 284 mg

## 28.  Chicken Zoodle Soup

**Preparation Time:** 15 minutes

**Cooking Time:** 35 minutes

**Servings:** 2

**Ingredients:**

- 1lb chopped cooked chicken
- 1lb spiralized zucchini
- 1 cup low sodium chicken soup
- 1 cup diced vegetables

Recipe:

1. Mix all the ingredients except the zucchini in your Instant Pot.

2. Cook on Stew for 35 minutes.

3. Release the pressure naturally.

4. Stir in the zucchini and allow to heat thoroughly.

**Nutrition:**

Calories: 250

Carbs: 5

Sugar: 0

Fat: 10

Protein: 40; GL: 1

## 29. Misto Quente

**Preparation Time:** 5 minutes

**Cooking Time:** 10 minutes

**Servings:** 4

**Ingredients:**

- 4 slices of bread without shell
- 4 slices of turkey breast
- 4 slices of cheese
- 2 tbsp. cream cheese
- 2 spoons of butter

**Directions:**

1. Preheat the air fryer. Set the timer of 5 minutes and the temperature to 200C.
2. Pass the butter on one side of the slice of bread, and on the other side of the slice, the cream cheese.
3. Mount the sandwiches placing two slices of turkey breast and two slices cheese between the breads, with the cream cheese inside and the side with butter.
4. Place the sandwiches in the basket of the air fryer. Set the timer of the air fryer for 5 minutes and press the power button.

**Nutrition**: Calories: 340 Fat: 15g Carbohydrates: 32g Protein: 15g Sugar: 0g Cholesterol: 0mg

# 30. Garlic Bread

**Preparation Time:** 10 minutes

**Cooking Time:** 15 minutes

**Servings:** 4-5

**Ingredients:**

- 2 stale French rolls
- 4 tbsp. crushed or crumpled garlic
- 1 cup of mayonnaise
- Powdered grated Parmesan
- 1 tbsp. olive oil

**Directions:**

1. Preheat the air fryer. Set the time of 5 minutes and the temperature to 2000C.
2. Mix mayonnaise with garlic and set aside.
3. Cut the baguettes into slices, but without separating them completely.
4. Fill the cavities of equals. Brush with olive oil and sprinkle with grated cheese.
5. Place in the basket of the air fryer. Set the timer to 10 minutes, adjust the temperature to 1800C and press the power button.

**Nutrition**: Calories: 340 Fat: 15g Carbohydrates: 32g Protein: 15g Sugar: 0g Cholesterol: 0mg

# 31. Bruschetta

**Preparation Time:** 5 minutes

**Cooking Time:** 10 minutes

**Servings:** 2

**Ingredients:**

- 4 slices of Italian bread
- 1 cup chopped tomato tea
- 1 cup grated mozzarella tea
- Olive oil
- Oregano, salt, and pepper
- 4 fresh basil leaves

**Directions:**

1. Preheat the air fryer. Set the timer of 5 minutes and the temperature to 2000C.
2. Sprinkle the slices of Italian bread with olive oil. Divide the chopped tomatoes and mozzarella between the slices. Season with salt, pepper, and oregano.
3. Put oil in the filling. Place a basil leaf on top of each slice.
4. Put the bruschetta in the basket of the air fryer being careful not to spill the filling. Set the timer of 5 minutes, set the temperature to 180C, and press the power button.
5. Transfer the bruschetta to a plate and serve.

**Nutrition**:

Calories: 434

Fat: 14g

Carbohydrates: 63g

Protein: 11g

Sugar: 8g

Cholesterol: 0mg

## 32. Cream Buns with Strawberries

**Preparation Time:** 10 minutes

**Cooking Time:** 12 minutes

**Servings:** 6

**Ingredients:**

- 240g all-purpose flour
- 50g granulated sugar
- 8g baking powder
- 1g of salt
- 85g chopped cold butter
- 84g chopped fresh strawberries
- 120 ml whipping cream
- 2 large eggs
- 10 ml vanilla extract
- 5 ml of water

**Directions:**

1. Sift flour, sugar, baking powder and salt in a large bowl. Put the butter with the flour with the use of a blender or your hands until the mixture resembles thick crumbs.
2. Mix the strawberries in the flour mixture. Set aside for the mixture to stand. Beat the whipping cream, 1 egg and the vanilla extract in a separate bowl.

3. Put the cream mixture in the flour mixture until they are homogeneous, and then spread the mixture to a thickness of 38 mm.
4. Use a round cookie cutter to cut the buns. Spread the buns with a combination of egg and water. Set aside
5. Preheat the air fryer, set it to 180C.
6. Place baking paper in the preheated inner basket.
7. Place the buns on top of the baking paper and cook for 12 minutes at 180C, until golden brown.

**Nutrition**: Calories: 150Fat: 14g Carbohydrates: 3g Protein: 11g Sugar: 8g Cholesterol: 0mg

## 33. Blueberry Buns

**Preparation Time:** 10 minutes

**Cooking Time:** 12 minutes

**Servings:** 6

**Ingredients:**

- 240g all-purpose flour
- 50g granulated sugar
- 8g baking powder
- 2g of salt
- 85g chopped cold butter
- 85g of fresh blueberries
- 3g grated fresh ginger
- 113 ml whipping cream
- 2 large eggs
- 4 ml vanilla extract
- 5 ml of water

**Directions:**

1. Put sugar, flour, baking powder and salt in a large bowl.
2. Put the butter with the flour using a blender or your hands until the mixture resembles thick crumbs.
3. Mix the blueberries and ginger in the flour mixture and set aside
4. Mix the whipping cream, 1 egg and the vanilla extract in a different container.

5. Put the cream mixture with the flour mixture until combined.
6. Shape the dough until it reaches a thickness of approximately 38 mm and cut it into eighths.
7. Spread the buns with a combination of egg and water. Set aside Preheat the air fryer set it to 180C.
8. Place baking paper in the preheated inner basket and place the buns on top of the paper. Cook for 12 minutes at 180C, until golden brown

**Nutrition**: Calories: 105 Fat: 1.64g Carbohydrates: 20.09gProtein: 2.43g Sugar: 2.1g Cholesterol: 0mg

## 34. Cauliflower Potato Mash

**Preparation Time:** 30 minutes **Servings:** 4

**Cooking Time:** 5 minutes

**Ingredients:**

- 2 cups potatoes, peeled and cubed
- 2 tbsp. butter
- ¼ cup milk
- 10 oz. cauliflower florets
- ¾ tsp. salt

**Directions:**

1. Add water to the saucepan and bring to boil.
2. Reduce heat and simmer for 10 minutes.
3. Drain vegetables well. Transfer vegetables, butter, milk, and salt in a blender and blend until smooth.
4. Serve and enjoy.

**Nutrition**: Calories 128 Fat 6.2 g, Sugar 3.3 g, Protein 3.2 g, Cholesterol 17 mg

## 35.  French toast in Sticks

**Preparation Time:** 5 minutes

**Cooking Time:** 10 minutes

**Servings:** 4

**Ingredients:**

- 4 slices of white bread, 38 mm thick, preferably hard
- 2 eggs
- 60 ml of milk
- 15 ml maple sauce
- 2 ml vanilla extract
- Nonstick Spray Oil
- 38g of sugar
- 3ground cinnamon
- Maple syrup, to serve
- Sugar to sprinkle

**Directions:**

1. Cut each slice of bread into thirds making 12 pieces. Place sideways
2. Beat the eggs, milk, maple syrup and vanilla.
3. Preheat the air fryer, set it to 175C.
4. Dip the sliced bread in the egg mixture and place it in the preheated air fryer. Sprinkle French toast generously with oil spray.
5. Cook French toast for 10 minutes at 175C. Turn the toast halfway through cooking.

6. Mix the sugar and cinnamon in a bowl.
7. Cover the French toast with the sugar and cinnamon mixture when you have finished cooking.
8. Serve with Maple syrup and sprinkle with powdered sugar

**Nutrition**: Calories 128 Fat 6.2 g, Carbohydrates 16.3 g, Sugar 3.3 g, Protein 3.2 g, Cholesterol 17 mg

# 36. Muffins Sandwich

**Preparation Time:** 2 minutes

**Cooking Time:** 10 minutes

**Servings:** 1

**Ingredients:**

- Nonstick Spray Oil
- 1 slice of white cheddar cheese
- 1 slice of Canadian bacon
- 1 English muffin, divided
- 15 ml hot water
- 1 large egg
- Salt and pepper to taste

**Directions:**

1. Spray the inside of an 85g mold with oil spray and place it in the air fryer.
2. Preheat the air fryer, set it to 160C.
3. Add the Canadian cheese and bacon in the preheated air fryer.
4. Pour the hot water and the egg into the hot pan and season with salt and pepper.
5. Select Bread, set to 10 minutes.
6. Take out the English muffins after 7 minutes, leaving the egg for the full time.
7. Build your sandwich by placing the cooked egg on top of the English muffing and serve

**Nutrition**:

Calories 400

Fat 26g

Carbohydrates 26g

Sugar 15 g

Protein 3 g

Cholesterol 155 mg

## 37.  Bacon BBQ

**Preparation Time:** 2 minutes

**Cooking Time:** 8 minutes

**Servings:** 2

**Ingredients:**

- 13g dark brown sugar
- 5g chili powder
- 1g ground cumin
- 1g cayenne pepper
- 4 slices of bacon, cut in half

**Directions:**

1. Mix seasonings until well combined.
2. Dip the bacon in the dressing until it is completely covered. Leave aside.
3. Preheat the air fryer, set it to 160C.
4. Place the bacon in the preheated air fryer
5. Select Bacon and press Start/Pause.

**Nutrition**: Calories: 1124 Fat: 72g Carbohydrates: 59g Protein: 49g Sugar: 11g Cholesterol: 77mg

# 38.  Stuffed French toast

**Preparation Time:** 4 minutes

**Cooking Time:** 10 minutes

**Servings:** 1

**Ingredients:**

- 1 slice of brioche bread,
- 64 mm thick, preferably rancid
- 113g cream cheese
- 2 eggs
- 15 ml of milk
- 30 ml whipping cream
- 38g of sugar
- 3g cinnamon
- 2 ml vanilla extract
- Nonstick Spray Oil
- Pistachios chopped to cover
- Maple syrup, to serve

**Directions:**

1. Preheat the air fryer, set it to 175C.
2. Cut a slit in the middle of the muffin.
3. Fill the inside of the slit with cream cheese. Leave aside.
4. Mix the eggs, milk, whipping cream, sugar, cinnamon, and vanilla extract.
5. Moisten the stuffed French toast in the egg mixture for 10 seconds on each side.

6. Sprinkle each side of French toast with oil spray.
7. Place the French toast in the preheated air fryer and cook for 10 minutes at 175C
8. Stir the French toast carefully with a spatula when you finish cooking.
9. Serve topped with chopped pistachios and acrid syrup.

**Nutrition**: Calories: 159Fat: 7.5g Carbohydrates: 25.2g Protein: 14g Sugar: 0g Cholesterol: 90mg

# 39. Scallion Sandwich

**Preparation Time:** 10 minutes

**Cooking Time:** 10 minutes

**Servings:** 1

**Ingredients:**

- 2 slices wheat bread
- 2 teaspoons butter, low fat
- 2 scallions, sliced thinly
- 1 tablespoon of parmesan cheese, grated
- 3/4 cup of cheddar cheese, reduced fat, grated

**Directions:**

1. Preheat the Air fryer to 356 degrees.
2. Spread butter on a slice of bread. Place inside the cooking basket with the butter side facing down.
3. Place cheese and scallions on top. Spread the rest of the butter on the other slice of bread Put it on top of the sandwich and sprinkle with parmesan cheese.
4. Cook for 10 minutes.

**Nutrition**: Calorie: 154Carbohydrate: 9g Fat: 2.5g Protein: 8.6g Fiber: 2.4g

# 40. Lean Lamb and Turkey Meatballs with Yogurt

**Preparation Time:** 10 minutes

**Servings:** 4

**Cooking Time:** 8 minutes

**Ingredients:**

- 1 egg white
- 4 ounces ground lean turkey
- 1 pound of ground lean lamb
- 1 teaspoon each of cayenne pepper, ground coriander, red chili pastes, salt, and ground cumin
- 2 garlic cloves, minced
- 1 1/2 tablespoons parsley, chopped
- 1 tablespoon mint, chopped
- 1/4 cup of olive oil

For the yogurt

- 2 tablespoons of buttermilk
- 1 garlic clove, minced
- 1/4 cup mint, chopped
- 1/2 cup of Greek yogurt, non-fat
- Salt to taste

**Directions:**

1. Set the Air Fryer to 390 degrees.

2. Mix all the ingredients for the meatballs in a bowl. Roll and mold them into golf-size round pieces. Arrange in the cooking basket. Cook for 8 minutes.
3. While waiting, combine all the ingredients for the mint yogurt in a bowl. Mix well.
4. Serve the meatballs with the mint yogurt. Top with olives and fresh mint.

5. **Nutrition**: Calorie: 154 Carbohydrate: 9g Fat: 2.5g Protein: 8.6g Fiber: 2.4g

# 41. Air Fried Section and Tomato

**Preparation Time:** 10 minutes

**Cooking Time:** 5 minutes

**Servings:** 2

**Ingredients:**

- 1 aubergine, sliced thickly into 4 disks
- 1 tomato, sliced into 2 thick disks
- 2 tsp. feta cheese, reduced fat
- 2 fresh basil leaves, minced
- 2 balls, small buffalo mozzarella, reduced fat, roughly torn
- Pinch of salt
- Pinch of black pepper

**Directions:**

1. Preheat Air Fryer to 330 degrees F.
2. Spray small amount of oil into the Air fryer basket. Fry aubergine slices for 5 minutes or until golden brown on both sides. Transfer to a plate.
3. Fry tomato slices in batches for 5 minutes or until seared on both sides.
4. To serve, stack salad starting with an aborigine base, buffalo mozzarella, basil

leaves, tomato slice, and 1/2-teaspoon feta cheese.

5. Top of with another slice of aborigine and 1/2 tsp. feta cheese. Serve.

**Nutrition**: Calorie: 140.3Carbohydrate: 26.6Fat: 3.4g Protein: 4.2g Fiber: 7.3g

## 42. Grain-Free Berry Cobbler

**Preparation Time:** 5 minutes

**Cooking Time:** 25 minutes

**Servings:** 10

**Ingredients:**

- 4 cups fresh mixed berries
- 1/2 cup ground flaxseed
- ¼ cup almond meal
- ¼ cup unsweetened shredded coconut
- 1/2 tablespoon baking powder
- 1 teaspoon ground cinnamon
- ¼ teaspoon salt
- Powdered stevia, to taste
- 6 tablespoons coconut oil

**Directions:**

1. Preheat the oven to 375F and lightly grease a 10-inch cast-iron skillet.
2. Spread the berries on the bottom of the skillet.
3. Whisk together the dry ingredients in a mixing bowl.
4. Cut in the coconut oil using a fork to create a crumbled mixture.
5. Spread the crumble over the berries and bake for 25 minutes until hot and bubbling.

6. Cool the cobbler for 5 to 10 minutes before serving.

**Nutrition**:

Calories 215

Total Fat 16.8g

Saturated Fat 10.4g

Total Carbs 13.1g

Net Carbs 6.7g

Protein 3.7g

Sugar 5.3g

Fiber 6.4g

Sodium 61mg

# Chapter 5. Dessert and Sweets

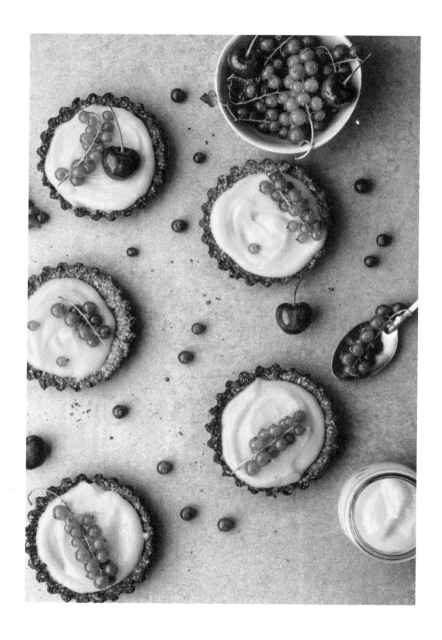

## 43. Frozen Lemon & Blueberry

**Preparation Time:** 5 minutes

**Cooking Time:** 10 minutes

**Servings:** 4

**Ingredients:**

- 6 cup fresh blueberries
- 8 sprigs fresh thyme
- ¾ cup light brown sugar
- 1 teaspoon lemon zest
- ¼ cup lemon juice
- 2 cups water

**Directions:**

1. Add blueberries, thyme and sugar in a pan over medium heat.
2. Cook for 6 to 8 minutes.
3. Transfer mixture to a blender.
4. Remove thyme sprigs.
5. Stir in the remaining ingredients.
6. Pulse until smooth.
7. Strain mixture and freeze for 1 hour.

**Nutrition:**

78 Calories; 20g Carbohydrate ; 3g Protein

# 44. Peanut Butter Choco Chip Cookies

**Preparation Time:** 5 minutes

**Cooking Time:** 10 minutes

**Servings:** 4

**Ingredients:**

- 1 egg
- ½ cup light brown sugar
- 1 cup natural unsweetened peanut butter
- Pinch salt
- ¼ cup dark chocolate chips

**Directions:**

1. Preheat your oven to 375 degrees F.
2. Mix egg, sugar, peanut butter, salt and chocolate chips in a bowl.
3. Form into cookies and place in a baking pan.
4. Bake the cookie for 10 minutes.
5. Let cool before serving.

**Nutrition:**

159 Calories

12g Carbohydrate

4.3g Protein

# 45. Watermelon Sherbet

**Preparation Time:** 5 minutes

**Cooking Time:** 3 minutes

**Servings:** 4

**Ingredients:**

- 6 cups watermelon, sliced into cubes
- 14 oz. almond milk
- 1 tablespoon honey
- ¼ cup lime juice
- Salt to taste

## Directions:

1. Freeze watermelon for 4 hours.
2. Add frozen watermelon and other ingredients in a blender.
3. Blend until smooth.
4. Transfer to a container with seal.
5. Seal and freeze for 4 hours.

## Nutrition:

132 Calories

24.5g Carbohydrate

3.1g Protein

# 46. Strawberry & Mango Ice Cream

**Preparation Time:** 5 minutes

**Cooking Time:** 10 minutes

**Servings:** 4

**Ingredients:**

- 8 oz. strawberries, sliced
- 12 oz. mango, sliced into cubes
- 1 tablespoon lime juice

**Directions:**

1. Add all ingredients in a food processor.
2. Pulse for 2 minutes.
3. Chill before serving.

**Nutrition:**

70 Calories

17.4g Carbohydrate

1.1g Protein

# 47. Sparkling Fruit Drink

**Preparation Time:** 5 minutes

**Cooking Time:** 10 minutes

**Servings:** 4

**Ingredients:**

- 8 oz. unsweetened grape juice
- 8 oz. unsweetened apple juice
- 8 oz. unsweetened orange juice
- 1 qt. homemade ginger ale
- Ice

**Directions:**

1. Makes 7 servings. Mix first 4 ingredients together in a pitcher.
2. Stir in ice cubes and 9 ounces of the beverage to each glass.
3. Serve immediately.

**Nutrition:**

60 Calories

1.1g Protein

# 48. Tiramisu Shots

**Preparation Time:** 5 minutes

**Cooking Time:** 10 minutes

**Servings:** 4

**Ingredients:**

- 1 pack silken tofu
- 1 oz. dark chocolate, finely chopped
- ¼ cup sugar substitute
- 1 teaspoon lemon juice
- ¼ cup brewed espresso
- Pinch salt
- 24 slices angel food cake
- Cocoa powder (unsweetened)

**Directions:**

1. Add tofu, chocolate, sugar substitute, lemon juice, espresso and salt in a food processor.
2. Pulse until smooth.
3. Add angel food cake pieces into shot glasses.
4. Drizzle with the cocoa powder.
5. Pour the tofu mixture on top.
6. Top with the remaining angel food cake pieces.
7. Chill for 30 minutes and serve.

**Nutrition**:

75 Calories

12g Carbohydrate

2.9g Protein

# 49. Ice Cream Brownie Cake

**Preparation Time:** 5 minutes

**Cooking Time:** 10 minutes

**Servings:** 4

**Ingredients:**

- Cooking spray
- 12 oz. no-sugar brownie mix
- ¼ cup oil
- 2 egg whites
- 3 tablespoons water
- 2 cups sugar-free ice cream

**Directions:**

1. Preheat your oven to 325 degrees F.
2. Spray your baking pan with oil.
3. Mix brownie mix, oil, egg whites and water in a bowl.
4. Pour into the baking pan.
5. Bake for 25 minutes.
6. Let cool.
7. Freeze brownie for 2 hours.
8. Spread ice cream over the brownie.
9. Freeze for 8 hours.

**Nutrition**:

198 Calories

33g Carbohydrate

3g Protein

# 50. Peanut Butter Cups

**Preparation Time:** 5 minutes

**Cooking Time:** 10 minutes

**Servings:** 4

**Ingredients:**

- 1 packet plain gelatin
- ¼ cup sugar substitute
- 2 cups nonfat cream
- ½ teaspoon vanilla
- ¼ cup low-fat peanut butter
- 2 tablespoons unsalted peanuts, chopped

**Directions:**

1. Mix gelatin, sugar substitute and cream in a pan.
2. Let sit for 5 minutes.
3. Place over medium heat and cook until gelatin has been dissolved.
4. Stir in vanilla and peanut butter.
5. Pour into custard cups. Chill for 3 hours.
6. Top with the peanuts and serve.

**Nutrition:**

171 Calories

21g Carbohydrate; 6.8g Protein

# Conclusion

Type 1 diabetes is all about being proactive, and being able to recognize when your blood sugars are getting too high and when they're too low. There are a lot of people with type 1 diabetes who don't know when their blood sugars are too high or too low or in what range they should be. Type II diabetes is the more common form of diabetes. It accounts for about 90 percent of diabetes cases. Type II diabetes usually occur because a person's body has lost the ability to produce insulin.

Type 1 diabetes occurs because the immune system destroys the insulin-producing cells of the pancreas. In the early stages of the disease, you may experience episodes of low blood sugar, called hypoglycemia, that can be dangerous if they occur frequently.

Having Type 1 diabetes will teach you a load of tough lessons. Only about ¼ of diabetics are Type 1. But I'm here to tell you, even though Type 1 is the most common type of diabetes, Type 2 diabetes can be almost as bad.

Being diagnosed with the disease will bring some major changes in your lifestyle. From the time you are diagnosed with it, it would always be a constant battle with food. You need to become a lot more careful with your food choices and the quantity that you ate. Every meal will feel like a major effort. You will be planning every day for the whole week, well in advance. Depending upon the type of food you ate, you have to keep checking your blood sugar levels. You may get used to taking long breaks between meals and staying away from snacks between dinner and breakfast.

Food would be treated as a bomb like it can go off at any time. According to an old saying, "When the body gets too hot, then your body heads straight to the kitchen."

Managing diabetes can be a very, very stressful ordeal. There will be many times that you will mark your glucose levels down on a piece of paper like you are plotting graph lines or something. You will mix your insulin shots up and then stress about whether or not you are giving yourself the right dosage. You will always be over-cautious because it involves a LOT of math and a really fine margin of error. But now, those days are gone!

With the help of technology and books, you can stock your kitchen with the right foods, like meal plans, diabetic friendly dishes, etc. You can get an app that will even do the work for you. You can also people-watch on the internet and find the know-how to cook and eat right; you will always be a few meals away from certain disasters, like a plummeting blood sugar level. Always carry some sugar in your pocket. You won't have to experience the pangs of hunger but if you are unlucky, you will have to ration your food and bring along some simple low-calorie snacks with you.

As you've reached the end of this book, you have gained complete control of your diabetes and this is just the beginning of your journey towards a better, healthier life.

Regardless of the length or seriousness of your diabetes, it can be managed! Take the information presented here and start with it!

CPSIA information can be obtained
at www.ICGtesting.com
Printed in the USA
BVHW011031280321
603594BV00002B/195